THE
EASY
10-Day Detox Diet
COOKBOOK

Chefon Press

THE EASY
10-Day Detox Diet
COOKBOOK

**Sugar Free, Whole Food, Dairy Free, Low-Carb Recipes
To Help Everyone Detox in Just 10 Days**

SARA S. WASABI

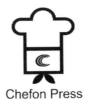

Chefon Press

DEDICATION

To all readers...

I know we haven't yet met each other. We have had only a glancing acquaintance because of this cookbook. However, even though we may never get a chance to meet each other, despite that, I am confident that we will often have fond thoughts of each other because of the benefits everyone will gain from this detox cookbook.

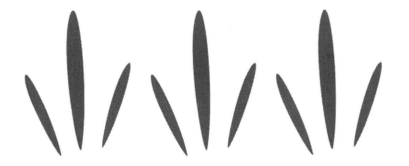

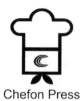

TABLE OF CONTENTS

DISCLAIMER

The information provided in this book is for educational purposes only. I am not a physician and this is not to be taken as medical advice or a recommendation to stop eating other foods. This book is based on my experiences and interpretations of the past and current research available. If you have any health issues or pre-existing conditions, please consult your doctor before implementing any of the information that is presented in this book. Results may vary from individual to individual. This book is for informational purposes only and the author or publisher does not accept any responsibilities for any liabilities or damages, real or perceived, resulting from the use of this information.

— 1 —

DETOXIFY FOR SUPERB HEALTH

"Lose weight, improve your health and take hold of genuine detox recipes that are supportive of your healthy detox goals for a 10-day program or even longer — that's what you'll get from the detox recipes in The Easy 10-Day Detox Diet Cookbook"

How about giving your body the ultimate cleanse? Or even better, how about accelerating your weight loss in just a few days? Well, if you're in for it, you'll be able to give your body just that. In the end your body will feel amazing and you will reap the superb health benefits. Whether you know it or not, a body detox is a proven and popular way to improve your overall health and to jump-start your weight loss. With the detox diet recipes in this book, you'll be able to give your body a well-deserved chance to attain optimum health.

Simply put, detoxification is a way of cleansing your system of "unwanted junk" or things that are slowing down your body's system, called toxins. While not all detox diets are created equal, there are still genuine detox diets that have gone through much scientific testing, research and thoughtful analysis. In essence, it is important that whichever detox program you decide to follow, you will be detoxifying in a gentle way that is supportive of your body, lifestyle and long term longevity.

− 2 −

WHY DO YOU NEED A DETOX?

We can all come to agree that we live in a very toxic world. We are exposed to different chemicals, pollutants and solvents on a daily basis through the food that we eat, the water that we drink, the air that we breathe and even other subtle toxins in our environment. The good news is that our bodies are really amazingly created to help us deal with and get rid of toxicity on a functional basis. However, our bodies are best supported with its daily detoxification functions if we help our body by eating the right foods and getting the right nutrients.

The liver is the main organ that is responsible for detoxification in the body and this organ needs to be well supported in order to get rid of the toxins that we are exposed to on a daily basis. Note that other organs are also involved in the detoxification process, such as the skin; however, the liver is the main organ of detoxification.

− 3 −

WHO CAN USE THIS COOKBOOK?

This is a versatile detox cookbook which contains genuine detox diet recipes that are **free from processed foods, sugars, dairy, starches, caffeine, beans and legumes, grains, alcohol and unhealthy oils**. These specially created recipes can be used on most (if not all) properly structured and nutrient-focused detox programs. Even more specifically, this cookbook can be used for:

- Persons that are looking for genuine 10-day Detox Diet recipes
- Persons that are on a smoothie or juice detox program and needs to continue eating healthy detox meals even afterwards
- Persons that are on any detox program that requires genuine detox recipes
- Persons seeking to jump-start their weight loss, burn belly fat or improve their overall health
- Persons looking for genuine detox recipes to help to clean their gut
- Persons looking to cleanse their system by simple eating healthy everyday meals

WHY DO YOU NEED THIS BOOK?

I believe that a healthy detox shouldn't come in a box or package. With this cookbook, you'll be able to prepare and eat healthy detox meals without the need to buy a detox in a box or package. Furthermore, this book will help you to experience sustained weight loss and good health by providing you with healthy detox recipes that can be used during and after your detox. Typically, in most detox programs, there is some degree of weight loss; however, the major challenge is actually maintaining permanent weight loss. There are persons who often regain the lost weight plus gain more weight at some point after their detox program has ended. With this detox cookbook you'll be able to eliminate that challenge and experience permanent weight loss.

In a nutshell, here are the benefits of using this detox cookbook:

- You'll be able to lose weight and keep it off
- You'll be able to ward off various sickness and disease
- You'll be able to choose and eat better foods
- You'll feel better , look better and live longer
- You'll improve your overall health
- You'll be able to detoxify your body naturally and without using harmful products or chemicals

– 4 –

5 COMMON DETOX MISTAKES YOU NEED TO AVOID

When it comes to detox, you wouldn't want to be derailed by a detox diet and then be forced to stop in the middle of the detox program. Your aim should be to detox successfully and to get the best desired health result from your detox efforts. Here are 5 very common detox mistakes that you should avoid so that you can get the most out of any structured detox program:

1. Avoid Going Cold Turkey
Some detox plans can be dangerous if you have certain lifestyle habits. Some of these habits may include, smoking or excessive use of alcohol, caffeine, sugars or other potentially harmful substances. Any dramatic shift in some of these harmful lifestyle habits into sudden detoxing may cause you to experience what is known as "withdrawal symptoms". With this said, your best bet is to slowly wean yourself off as many toxins as possible before starting your detox. For example you may think about giving up one habit per day, such as alcohol, processed foods or sugars and you should continue doing this up to the day that you've decided to actually start your detox program.

2. Avoid Starving Yourself
For many, the first thing that comes to mind when they think of

"detox" is that it is all about starving yourself. This could not be further from the truth. There is absolutely no need to deprive yourself of calories while you are on a detox program. Isn't that a relief? All you need to do is start eating smarter. Smarter eating means that you should avoid processed foods, dairy, artificial ingredients, sugars, starches, legumes and unhealthy fats. On a properly structured detox program, you should incorporate plenty of healthy detox whole foods such as non-starchy vegetables, low-sugar fruits, healthy nuts and seeds (no peanuts) and lean protein.

3. Avoid Drinking Little Water
In general, sufficient water intake is important for good health. On a detox program, sufficient water intake is of paramount importance. By proper hydration you will be able to minimize or alleviate common detox symptoms such as headaches, fatigue, diarrhea, crankiness, nausea and vomiting. Water hydration will also help your body to flush out toxins from your body's tissues during the detox. In light of this, as you go through your detox program, an important question that you need to ask yourself is: Am I drinking enough water? You should drink much water between meals and consume at least 64 fluid ounces on a daily basis.

4. Avoid Lack of Knowledge About The Detox Program
Not all detox programs are for everyone. Because of this, it is a good idea to educate yourself as much as possible in order to ensure that a particular detox program can work for you. Some detox programs may be designed for weight loss while others are designed to specifically remove toxins from the body. Many scientists and doctors such as Dr. Michael Smith of Carolinas Natural Health Center have come to agree that the best detox plans are the ones that do not restrict calories and also has a balance of nutrients. Apart from choosing wisely, it is always a good idea to consult your doctor before you start any kind of detox program.

5. Avoid Having a Food Blast Right After Your Detox

After the completion of your detox program, instead of going back to your pre-detox lifestyle or eating habits, it is best to continue incorporating detox foods into your diet at least once weekly. Remember that you want the best results and overall good health from your detox. The detox recipes in this cookbook are specially created to help you to stay on track with healthy detox recipes that can be used during and after your detox.

BENEFITS OF A HEALTHY DETOX DIET

On a healthy detox diet your aim should be to eat alkaline foods, foods that are easy to digest, anti-inflammatory foods and foods that can cleanse your system. Here follows a list of some benefits of detoxifying your body. Please note this is not a conclusive list of benefits that you will get from detoxifying your body:

- Speedy weight loss
- Decreased belly fat
- Regularized bowel movements
- Improved digestion
- Decreased bloating and acid reflux
- Increased energy levels
- Improvement in mood and overall feeling of well-being
- Improved liver functions
- Overall increased of vitality and longevity

COME ON, LET'S DETOX

With *The Easy 10-Day Detox Diet Cookbook* you'll be able to take hold of genuine detox recipes that are healthy and supportive of your healthy detox goals.

Whichever recipe you choose from this special collection of detox diet recipes, it's totally up to you. Just get your ingredients and follow the directions—it is surprisingly simple. In some cases, you may make your own ingredient substitutions and tweak the recipes here and there based on your preferences or individual situations.

Now, it's time to try your hand at creating healthy and easy detox meals using these specially developed recipes. Happy detoxing!

– 6 –

DETOX BREAKFAST RECIPES

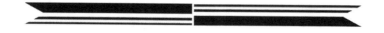

Green Detox Smoothie

This smoothie contains flaxseeds and has a wonderful and nutrient-rich combo of healthy greens, berries and cinnamon.

Servings: 2
Preparation Time: 10 minutes

¼ Cucumber, peeled and sliced
2 cups Spinach, trimmed and chopped
½ Stalk Celery
1 cup Frozen Mixed Berries
2 tablespoons Flaxseeds, (optional: presoak for 30 minutes or overnight)
2 cups Water
1 teaspoon Ground Cinnamon
6 Ice Cubes

Directions:

1. In a blender, add all ingredients and blend until well combined and smooth.
2. Serve immediately.

Pumpkin Dream Smoothie

This smoothie gives the taste of a pumpkin pie in a glass. This unique and healthy smoothie is rich and flavorful.

Servings: 2
Preparation Time: 5 minutes

---

6 tablespoons Homemade Pumpkin Puree
1 tablespoon Chia Seeds, (optional: presoak for 30 minutes or overnight)
1 tablespoon Pumpkin Seeds, (optional: presoak for 30 minutes or overnight)
1 teaspoon Ground Cinnamon
1/8 teaspoon Nutmeg, grated freshly
1 tablespoon Almond Butter
1½ cups unsweetened Almond Milk
6 Ice Cubes

Directions:

1. In a blender, add all ingredients and pulse until well combined and smooth.
2. Serve immediately.

Green Strawberry Ginger Smoothie

Start your day in a great way by blending this healthy smoothie for breakfast. With a combination of spinach and strawberries, this smoothie is bursting with vitamins and antioxidant goodness.

Servings: 1
Preparation Time: 5 minutes

---

6 Large Spinach Leaves
1½ cups Fresh Strawberries
2 teaspoons Fresh Ginger, grated
1 tablespoon Fresh Lime Juice
½ cup Water
1 cup Ice Cubes

Directions:

1. In a blender, add all ingredients and pulse until well combined and smooth.
2. Serve immediately.

Blueberry Appeal Smoothie

This yummy smoothie combines the sweetness of apples and almond milk to make a quick and easy smoothie treat.

Servings: 1
Preparation Time: 5 minutes

1 cup unsweetened Almond Milk
1 cup frozen Blueberries
2 teaspoons Cinnamon Powder
2 tablespoons Pecan Butter

Directions:

1. In a blender, add all ingredients and pulse till well combined and smooth.
2. Serve immediately.

Blackberry Coco Greens Smoothie

*This healthy but incredibly delicious **smoothie** is made with blackberries and nutritious dandelion greens. Enjoy every sip.*

Servings: 2
Preparation Time: 10 minutes

---

1 cup frozen Blackberries
1 cup Water
½ tablespoon of your favorite Nut Butter (except peanut butter)
½ cups unsweetened Coconut Milk
1 cup Dandelion Greens
6 Ice Cubes

Directions:

1. In a blender, add all ingredients and pulse until well combined and smooth.
2. Serve immediately.

Raspberry Cinnamon Smoothie

This summer smoothie is a great hit for a healthy breakfast. At the same time it is so refreshing and delicious too.

Servings: 2
Preparation Time: 10 minutes

---

1 cup frozen Raspberries
2 tablespoons Flaxseeds, (optional: presoak for 30 minutes or overnight)
2 tablespoons Almond Butter
5 Large Lettuce Leaves
1½ cups Water
Pinch of Ground Cinnamon

Directions:

1. In a blender, add all ingredients and blend until well combined and smooth.
2. Serve immediately

Beet Detox Smoothie

Beets are among the best natural liver detox foods around. With this beet detox smoothie, you'll be able to help body further in its natural detoxification process.

Serves: 2
Prep Time: 10 minutes

½ cup filtered Water
1 cup frozen Raspberries
1 small Beet, ends trimmed and roughly chopped
¼ of an Avocado, peeled, pitted and cubed
1 Celery Stalk, roughly chopped
1 teaspoon fresh Lemon or Lime Juice
½ tablespoon Coconut oil (optional)
2 large Ice Cubes

Directions:

1. In a high-speed blender, add all ingredients and blend until well combined and smooth.
2. Serve immediately

Note: Add all ingredients into a high-speed blender and blend on high until smooth. Adjust sweetness only if desired, adding an apple or liquid sweetener to taste if needed.

Fresh Berry Garden Smoothie

This is a quick and delicious breakfast option. This smoothie is a really earthy and healthy breakfast smoothie.

Servings: 2
Preparation Time: 10 minutes

---

1 cup of your favorite frozen Berries
½ cup Baby Spinach
½ Celery Stalk, chopped
¼ of an Avocado, peeled, pitted and chopped
1-inch Fresh Ginger Piece, grated
1 teaspoon Sesame Seeds, (optional: presoak for 30 minutes or overnight)
½ cup Water
½ cup unsweetened Almond Milk

Directions:

1. In a blender, add all ingredients and blend until well combined and smooth.
2. Serve immediately

Green Berry Smoothie

This green berry smoothie is packed with antioxidants and essential vitamins and minerals. This is considered a low sugar smoothie which has sugar mainly from the blueberries and raspberries.

Serves: 2
Prep Time: 10 minutes

---

1 cup Water
1 cup Kale, washed and torn
½ of an Avocado
½ cup Wild Blueberries, fresh
½ cup Raspberries, fresh
½ cup Ice Cubes

Directions:

1. Place the water in the blender first then add in the remaining ingredients.
2. Blend until you achieve your desired smoothie consistency. In order to adjust the consistency, add a little more water if necessary.

Gingery Blackberry Bliss Smoothie

By using spinach in this smoothie, it will give a very nice consistency and powerful nutrients when combined with the other ingredients.

Serves: 2
Prep Time: 10 minutes

---

1 cup Blackberries, fresh
½ cup Spinach, washed and torn
½ cup Unsweetened Almond Milk (add more to adjust consistency)
½ tablespoon Extra-virgin Coconut Butter
2 teaspoons Ginger, freshly peeled and grated
1 cup Ice Cubes

Directions:

1. Place the almond milk in the blender first then add in the remaining ingredients.
2. Blend until you achieve your desired smoothie consistency. In order to adjust the consistency, add more water if necessary.

Raspberry Pecan Smoothie

This smoothie uses a healthy combination of fresh raspberries which are loaded with essential vitamins, minerals and fiber. It also uses pecan butter which has healthy fat and isn't very sweet.

***Serves:** 2*
***Prep Time:** 10 minutes*

---

1 cup Fresh Raspberries (you may substitute with your favorite berries)
4 tablespoons Unsweetened Almond Milk
2 tablespoons Natural Smooth Pecan Butter
1 cup Ice Cubes

Directions:

1. Place the almond milk in the blender first then add in the remaining ingredients.
2. Blend until you achieve your desired smoothie consistency. In order to adjust the consistency, add more almond milk if necessary.

Creamy Blackberry Smoothie

Blackberry Choi smoothie is rich in antioxidants, healthy fats and fiber. It has no sugar added except for that which comes from the blackberries and is great for satisfying hunger pangs.

Serves: 1-2
Prep Time: 10 minutes

---

1 cup Water
1 cup frozen Blackberries (ensure that these are free from added sugar)
½ ripe Avocado
½ cup Pak Choi

Directions:

1. Place all ingredients into your blender and process until a smooth consistency is achieved or for about a minute.
2. Pour in a glass and serve.

Deluxe Almond Smoothie

This healthy low carb smoothie is a great almond treat which is made very creamy with a slice of avocado. Drink this healthy glass of smoothie and boost your energy levels.

Serves: 1
Prep Time: 10 minutes

---

1 cup unsweetened Almond Milk
½ cup frozen Cranberries (ensure that these are free from added sugar)
1 slice ripe Avocado
2 tablespoons natural Almond Butter
1 tablespoon Pumpkin Seeds
2 Walnuts
½ cup Ice Cubes

Directions:

1. Place all ingredients into your blender and process until smooth or for about a minute.
2. Pour in a glass and serve.

Cucumber Berry Smoothie

This cucumber smoothie recipe is great for the skin and kidneys. Detox your body while you also enjoy every sip of this fiber-rich smoothie.

Serves: 2
Prep Time: 10 minutes

---

2 large Cucumbers, washed, peeled and cut into chunks
1 cup unsweetened Almond Milk
1 cup frozen Raspberries (ensure that these are free from added sugar)
½ teaspoon Cinnamon Powder (optional)

Directions:

1. Place all ingredients into your blender and process until smooth consistency is achieved or for about a minute.
2. Pour in a glass and serve.

Super Detox Smoothie

This is an extremely healthy smoothie for detoxifying the body and it has no added sugar. Based on its taste, this smoothie is not for the faint of heart, however, it is loaded with essential vitamins and minerals to boost your overall health and also detoxify your body. You'll know you're drinking something healthy with every sip. Try it!

Serves: 2
Prep Time: 10 minutes

---

1 large handful of Kale or Spinach
½ of a Bell Pepper
¾ of an Avocado
2 cloves Garlic
2 ripe Tomatoes
2 cups of Water

Directions:

1. Place all ingredients into your blender and process until smooth consistency is achieved or for about a minute.
2. Pour in a glass and serve.

Strawberry Chia Shake

This is a protein packed recipe of a yummy strawberry shake.
This shake will have a mild nutty flavor and a very mild taste too.

Servings: 2
Preparation Time: 5 minutes

---

2 cups Frozen Strawberries, hulled
2 tablespoons Chia Seeds, (optional: presoak for 30 minutes or overnight)
1½ cups Unsweetened Almond Milk
2 tablespoons Almond Butter
½ cup Ice Cubes

Directions:

1. In a blender, add all ingredients and pulse until smooth and creamy.
2. Serve immediately.

Pecan Avocado Shake

This is another quick and delicious breakfast option. This avocado shake may become one of your favorites.

Servings: 2
Preparation Time: 5 minutes

½ of an Avocado, peeled, pitted and sliced
2 cups unsweetened Almond Milk
½ cup frozen Strawberries
1 tablespoon Pecan Butter
½ tablespoon Pumpkin Seeds, (optional: presoak for 30 minutes or overnight)
½ cup Ice Cubes

Directions:

1. In a blender, add all ingredients and pulse until smooth and creamy.
2. Serve immediately.

Very Almond Shake

This is a quick and easy option for breakfast. This shake is a very healthy and fulfilling.

Servings: 2
Preparation Time: 5 minutes

¾ cup Almonds, chopped, (optional: presoak for 30 minutes or overnight)
1 cup frozen Strawberries, hulled
1½ cups unsweetened Almond Milk
2 tablespoons Almond Butter
½ cup Ice Cubes

Directions:

1. In a blender, add all ingredients and pulse till smooth and creamy.
2. Serve immediately.

Tofu Berry Shake

With tofu in this smoothie, it adds protein and gives a more silky touch. Enjoy this for your silky morning treat.

Servings: 2
Preparation Time: 10 minutes

¾ cup Soft Tofu
2 cups Frozen Raspberries, hulled
1 cup unsweetened Almond Milk
2 tablespoons hemp seeds, (optional: presoak for 30 minutes or overnight)
½ cup Ice Cubes

Directions:

1. In a blender, add all ingredients and pulse until well combined and smooth.
2. Serve immediately.

– 7 –

LUNCH DETOX RECIPES

Grilled Veggie Salad

This unique salad is quite colorful with the veggies and can be a tasty change from ordinary salads. Garnish this salad with chopped scallions.

Servings: 2
Preparation Time: 20 minutes

For Salad:

1 Green Bell Pepper, halved and seeded
1 Red Bell Pepper, halved and seeded
1 Medium Zucchini, sliced ½-inch thickness
1 cup Grape Tomatoes
1 Red Onion, cut into 8 wedges
1 tablespoon Extra Virgin Olive Oil
Sea Salt and Black Pepper, to taste
2 tablespoons Black Olives, pitted and sliced
2 tablespoons Fresh Mint Leaves, chopped

For Vinaigrette:

1 tablespoon Balsamic Vinegar
1 teaspoon Fresh Lemon Juice
1 tablespoon Extra Virgin Olive Oil
1 Garlic Clove, minced
Sea Salt and Black Pepper, to taste

Directions:

1. Preheat the grill to medium-high heat, Grease the grill grate.
2. In a large serving bowl, add bell peppers, zucchini, tomatoes, onion, oil, salt and black pepper and toss to coat well. Place bell peppers and onion on grill grate and grill for 10 minutes. Remove bell peppers from grill. Flip the onion. Place zucchini on grill grate and grill for 5 minutes. Remove onion and flip the side of zucchini. Place tomatoes and grill for 5 minutes. Peel and slice the bell peppers.
3. In a bowl, add vinaigrette ingredients and beat until well combined.
4. In a large serving bowl, add grilled vegetables, olives, mint and mix together. Pour vinaigrette and toss to coat well.

Spinach Salad with Salmon

This is a real cinch to make salad which can be a wonderful light lunch for all and surely keep you going for hours. Top with freshly grated lemon zest.

Servings: 2
Preparation Time: 15 minutes

For Salad:

6-ounces Smoked Salmon
2 Plum Tomatoes, chopped
1 cup Fresh Baby Spinach Leaves
1 Avocado, peeled, pitted and chopped

For Vinaigrette:

2½ tablespoons Balsamic Vinegar
2 tablespoons Extra Virgin Olive Oil
2 tablespoons Fresh Lemon Juice
Sea Salt and Black Pepper, to taste

Directions:

1. In a large serving bowl, add all salad ingredients and mix.
2. In another small bowl, add vinaigrette ingredients and beat until well combined.

3. Pour vinaigrette over salad, toss to coat well and serve.

Roasted Bell Pepper & Tomato Soup

This soup has a very satisfying and delicious taste. It could turn out to be an instant hit for your whole family. You may drizzle this soup with some fresh lime juice for a little tangy touch.

Servings: 4
Preparation Time: 15 minutes
Cooking Time: 45 minutes

---

1 Large Orange Bell Pepper, seeded and quartered
1 Large Red Bell Pepper, seeded and quartered
2¼ pounds Plum Tomatoes, halved
1 Yellow Onion, sliced thinly
4 Large Garlic Cloves, peeled
1 tablespoon Olive Oil
Sea Salt and Black Pepper, to taste
1 teaspoon Fresh Thyme Leaves
2 tablespoons Fresh Oregano Leaves
2 cups Low Sodium Vegetable Broth

Directions:

1. Preheat the oven to 450 degrees F. Line a large baking sheet with foil paper.
2. Place bell peppers, tomatoes, onion and garlic in prepared baking sheet. Drizzle with olive oil and then sprinkle with salt and black pepper. Bake for about 40 minutes, flipping occasionally. Remove from oven

and keep aside to cool it.

3. In a food processor, add roasted vegetables, herbs and broth and pulse in batches until smooth. Transfer the soup in a pan.

4. Cook, stirring occasionally for about 4 to 5 minutes or until heated completely. Season with desired salt and black pepper. Serve hot.

Spicy Turkey & Avocado Soup

This is an excellent soup with spicy touch. Avocado brings an exotic change and creaminess in this turkey soup. Garnish with freshly grated lime zest.

Servings: 4
Preparation Time: 10 minutes
Cooking Time: 30 minutes

---

3 cups Low Sodium Vegetable Broth
1½ cups Cooked Turkey, shredded
1 Medium Yellow Onion, chopped
1 Garlic Clove, minced
1 Green Chile, chopped
1 tablespoon Fresh Lime Juice
¼ teaspoon Ground Cumin
¼ teaspoon Ground Coriander
¼ teaspoon Cayenne Pepper
Sea Salt and Black Pepper, to taste
½ Medium Avocado, peeled, pitted and chopped
3 tablespoons Fresh Basil, chopped

Directions:

1. In a large soup pan, add all ingredients except avocado and basil and bring to a boil on medium-high heat.
2. Reduce the heat to low and simmer for about 12 to

15 minutes.
3. Stir in avocado and simmer for 12 to 15 minutes.
4. Stir in basil and season with salt and black pepper if required.

Chicken & Veggie Soup

This is one classically comforting chicken soup. This classic soup is not only tasty but also healthy too. Serve with a toping of fresh parsley leaves.

Servings: 4
Preparation Time: 20 minutes
Cooking Time: 40 minutes

---

2 teaspoons Olive Oil
1 Medium Yellow Onion, chopped
3 Garlic Cloves, minced
4 Carrots, peeled and chopped
2 Stalks Celery, sliced
2 pounds Boneless, Skinless Chicken Breasts, cut into bite sized pieces
6 cups Low Sodium Vegetable Broth
½ teaspoon Dried Rosemary, crushed
Sea Salt and Black Pepper, to taste

Directions:

1. In a large soup pan, heat oil on medium heat. Add onion and sauté for 4 to 5 minutes.
2. Add garlic, carrots and celery and cook, stirring for 4 to 5 minutes.

3. Add chicken and broth and bring to a boil. Reduce the heat to low. Simmer for 25 to 30 minutes while stirring occasionally.
4. Stir in dried rosemary and season with salt and black pepper if required.

Go-Easy Garlicky Shrimp

This simple and delicious recipe has a classic garlicky touch. Shrimp lovers will give another try to this delicious shrimp recipe soon. Serve with fresh lime wedges.

Servings: 2
Preparation Time: 10 minutes
Cooking Time: 7 minutes

---

2 teaspoons Coconut Oil
½ pound Shrimp, deveined
3 Garlic Cloves, minced
Sea Salt and Black Pepper, to taste
Pinch of Red Pepper Flakes

Directions:

1. In a skillet, heat oil on medium heat. Add shrimps and garlic. Sprinkle or season the shrimp with salt, black pepper and the pinch of red pepper flakes.
2. Cook for about 6 to 7 minutes or until done completely.

Roasted Veggie Combo

This dish is so easy to make and a great way to roast green beans and bell peppers. It will be a solid addition to your menu. Serve these roasted veggies with broiled fish.

Servings: 2
Preparation Time: 15 minutes
Cooking Time: 15 minutes

---

1 pound Green Beans, trimmed and halved
1 Small Orange Bell Pepper, seeded and sliced in thin strips
1 Small Red Bell Pepper, seeded and sliced in thin strips
1 tablespoon Coconut Oil, melted
1 tablespoon Ginger, minced
1 tablespoon Garlic, minced
1 teaspoon Dried Rosemary, crushed
Sea Salt and Black Pepper, to taste

Directions:

1. Preheat the oven to 450 degrees F. Line a large baking sheet with foil paper.
2. In a large bowl, add all ingredients and toss to coat well. Place the veggie mixture in prepared baking sheet in a single layer.
3. Roast for about 15 minutes or until tender crisp.

Gingery Chicken Mushroom

This is definitely a winning combination for a wonderful lunch. It is quick to prepare but at the same time it is also rich in taste. Serve with tossed salad.

Servings: 2
Preparation Time: 15 minutes
Cooking Time: 15 minutes

---

2 teaspoons Coconut Oil
1 Medium Yellow Onion, chopped
6 Garlic Cloves, minced
1 tablespoon Fresh Ginger, minced
2 (4-ounces) Boneless, Skinless Chicken Breasts, cut into ½-inch strips
1 tablespoon Balsamic Vinegar
½ cup Unsweetened Coconut Milk
Pinch of Red Pepper Flakes
1½ cups Button Mushrooms, sliced thinly
¼ cup Fresh Thyme, chopped
Sea Salt and Black Pepper, to taste

Directions:

1. In a large skillet, heat oil on medium-high heat. Add in chopped onion, garlic and ginger and allow to sauté for about 3 to 4 minutes.
2. Add chicken and cook for 3 to 4 minutes. Add

vinegar, milk and red pepper flakes. Bring to a boil and reduce the heat to medium-low.

3. Cook for 3 to 4 minutes. Add mushrooms and thyme and cook for 2 to 3 minutes.
4. Season with salt and black pepper and serve hot.

Chicken & Tomato Skewers

This is a quick and amazingly delicious dish. These skewers make an easy nibble that may fit in at your buffet party. Serve with orange salad or as desired.

Servings: 2
Preparation Time: 10 minutes
Cooking Time: 8 minutes

1/3 cup Fresh Cilantro Leaves
2 tablespoons Almonds, chopped
1 Small Garlic Clove, chopped
1 tablespoon Coconut Oil, melted
Sea Salt and Black Pepper, to taste
2 (4-ounces) Boneless, Skinless Chicken Breasts, cubed
8 Grapes Tomatoes

Directions:

1. In a blender, add all ingredients except chicken and tomatoes and pulse until pureed. Transfer the mixture in a large bowl. Add chicken and coat generously. Cover and refrigerate to marinate for at least 2 hours.
2. Preheat the grill to medium heat. Grease the grill grate.
3. Thread the chicken cubes and tomatoes evenly on pre-soaked skewers.

4. Grill for about 3 to 4 minutes per side.

Herbed Roasted Turkey & Veggies

These classic and delish flavors combine together nicely with this family-pleasing roasted turkey. Make this meal to please your family and friends. Enjoy with fresh greens.

Servings: 2
Preparation Time: 20 minutes
Cooking Time: 40 minutes

½ teaspoon Onion Powder
½ teaspoon Dried Oregano, crushed
½ teaspoon Dried Basil, crushed
½ teaspoon Dried Dill, crushed
Sea Salt and Black Pepper, to taste
1 Large Red Onion, cut into wedges
3 Celery Ribs, sliced
2 cups Fresh Baby Carrots
3 teaspoons Coconut Oil, melted and divided
2 Skinless Turkey Breast Tenderloins

Directions:

1. Preheat the oven to 425 degrees F. Line a roasting pan with foil paper.
2. In a bowl, mix together onion powder, herbs, salt and black pepper. Transfer half of herb mixture in a large bowl. Add vegetables and 2 teaspoons of oil and toss to coat well. Place the veggie mixture in prepared

roasting pan. Roast the veggie mixture for about 15 minutes.

3. Meanwhile in a bowl, place turkey tenderloins. Add remaining herb mixture and oil and coat over turkey tenderloins.
4. Remove baking pan from oven. Place the turkey tenderloins in the center of pan, moving vegetables to the sides. Roast for about 20 to 25 minutes.

Salmon & Asparagus Parcels

This is a guaranteed winner recipe on any party table! This is a fool proof recipe for baking the fish. Serve with fresh lime wedges.

Servings: 2
Preparation Time: 20 minutes
Cooking Time: 40 minutes

---

2 (4-ounces) Salmon Fillets
1 Small Plum Tomato, seeded and chopped
1 Small Red Onion, sliced thinly
1 Garlic Clove, chopped finely
1 tablespoon Fresh Lime Juice
Sea Salt and Black Pepper, to taste
1 Fresh Rosemary Sprig
½ pound Asparagus, trimmed
1 teaspoon Coconut Oil, melted

Directions:

1. Preheat the oven to 400 degrees Fahrenheit. Grease a baking sheet.
2. Place two foil papers on top of each other. Grease with cooking spray. Place a fish fillet over foil paper. Place half of tomato and onion over fish. Drizzle with lime juice. Sprinkle with salt and black pepper. Place rosemary sprig and asparagus

on top. Drizzle with oil.
3. Fold the short ends of foil to make a packet. Make another parcel in the same way.
4. Arrange both of the packets in prepared baking sheet. Bake for about 25 minutes.

Nutty Cauliflower Delight

This super healthy, delicious and spicy dish is also a good source of vitamin C. The combination of spices gives this baked cauliflower an excellent touch. Serve with fresh baby spinach leaves.

Servings: 2
Preparation Time: 10 minutes
Cooking Time: 25 minutes

---

1 Medium Head Cauliflower, cut into florets
1 teaspoon Olive Oil
1 teaspoon Coriander Seeds
1 teaspoon Cumin Seeds
1 teaspoon Red Pepper Flakes, crushed
Sea Salt and Black Pepper, to taste
¼ cup Almonds, chopped
1 tablespoon Fresh Lemon Juice
1 teaspoon Lemon Zest, grated freshly

Directions:

1. Preheat the oven to 400 degrees F.
2. In a pan of boiling water, add cauliflower and boil for about 2 to 3 minutes. Remove from heat and drain well.
3. In an oven proof skillet, heat oil on medium-low heat. Add coriander, cumin, red pepper flakes and

sauté for 1 minute. Add cauliflower and almonds. Sprinkle with salt and black pepper and sauté for 4 to 5 minutes. Stir in lemon juice and zest and cook for 1 minute more.

4. Remove the skillet from stove and transfer into oven. Bake for 15 minutes.

Chicken Broccoli Stir Fry

This beautifully colored and healthy dish will amuse all at the dining table. Broccoli and chicken combines greatly in this dish. Top with chopped walnuts.

Servings: 2
Preparation Time: 10 minutes
Cooking Time: 25 minutes

1½ teaspoons Olive Oil
2 (4-ounces) Boneless, Skinless Chicken Breasts, cubed
½ teaspoon Fresh Ginger, minced
1 teaspoon Fresh Garlic, minced
2 cups Broccoli Florets
1 Small Red Bell Pepper, seeded and sliced
1 Small Orange Bell Pepper, seeded and sliced
Pinch of Red Pepper Flakes, crushed
Sea Salt and Black Pepper, to taste
½ cup Low Sodium Vegetable Broth

Directions:
1. In a nonstick skillet, heat oil on medium-high heat. Add chicken and stir fry for 3 to 4 minutes. Add ginger and garlic and stir fry for 1 minute more.
2. Add broccoli and bell peppers. Sprinkle with red pepper flakes, salt and black pepper. Pour broth and bring to a boil.
3. Reduce the heat to medium-low. Allow to cook for 8

to 10 minutes.

Turkey & Cabbage Fiesta

This great tasting combination of turkey, tomato and cabbage makes a hearty and filling dish. Top with freshly chopped parsley.

Servings: 2
Preparation Time: 10 minutes
Cooking Time: 30 minutes

1teaspoons Olive Oil
1 Shallot, chopped finely
2 Garlic Cloves, minced
½ pound Lean Ground Turkey
1¼ cups Tomatoes, chopped
½ Head Cabbage, chopped
½ cup Low Sodium Vegetable Broth
Sea Salt and Black Pepper, to taste

Directions:

1. In a nonstick skillet, heat oil on medium heat. Add shallot and garlic and sauté for 3 to 4 minutes.
2. Add turkey and cook for 5 to 6 minutes. Stir in cabbage and tomatoes and reduce the heat to low. Add broth, cover and simmer for 20 minutes or until done completely.
3. Season with salt and black pepper and serve hot.

Curried Shrimp with Orange

This shrimp curry will have you out of the kitchen in no time. The nice sweetness from the orange compliments the heat of spices very well.

Servings: 2
Preparation Time: 15 minutes
Cooking Time: 10 minutes

¼ teaspoon Curry Powder
¼ teaspoon Ground Cumin
Garlic Powder, to taste
Ginger Powder, to taste
Pinch of Cayenne Pepper
½ pound Shrimps, shelled
½ cup Low Sodium Vegetable Broth
½ cup Onion, chopped finely
2 cups Cabbage, shredded finely
Sea Salt and Black Pepper, to taste
2 tablespoons Fresh Lemon Juice
2 Oranges, peeled, seeded and sectioned

Directions:
1. In a bowl, add all spices and mix. Add shrimp and coat with spice mixture evenly. Keep aside for 10 minutes.
2. In a large skillet, add broth on medium-high heat. Add shrimp mixture, onion and cabbage and bring to

a boil.

3. Reduce the heat to low. Cover and simmer for about 10 minutes or until done completely. Season with salt and black pepper if required.

4. Transfer the shrimp mixture in a serving plate. Drizzle with lemon juice. Top with orange and serve.

Sautéed Garlicky Mushrooms

All mushrooms blend together with garlic and vinegar in this dish very well. Serve with fresh veggie salad.

Servings: 2
Preparation Time: 15 minutes
Cooking Time: 10 minutes

1teaspoon Extra Virgin Olive Oil
1½ cups Crimini Mushrooms, sliced thinly
1½ cups Shitake Mushrooms, sliced thinly
1½ cups Portobello Mushrooms, sliced thinly
2 Garlic Cloves, minced
2 tablespoons Fresh Cilantro, chopped
1 tablespoon Balsamic Vinegar
Sea Salt and Black Pepper, to taste
1 tablespoon Pecans, toasted and chopped

Directions:
1. In a large skillet, heat oil on medium-high heat. Next, add in the mushrooms and sauté for about 3 minutes. Add in garlic and sauté for 4 to 5 minutes.
2. Stir in cilantro and vinegar and cook for 1 to 2 minutes more.
3. Season with salt and black pepper. Remove from heat, top with pecans and serve.

Grilled Tangy Chicken with Roasted Tomatoes

This grilled chicken recipe is truly bursting with the flavors of fresh lime. This robust marinade adds a refreshing touch to the chicken. Garnish with fresh lime zest.

Servings: 2
Preparation Time: 15 minutes
Cooking Time: 20 minutes

For Grilled Chicken:

½ teaspoon Extra Virgin Olive Oil
1 Garlic Clove, minced
½ tablespoon Fresh Lime Juice
½ tablespoon Lime Zest, grated freshly
2 (4-ounces) Boneless, Skinless Chicken Thighs
Sea Salt and Black Pepper, to taste

For Tomatoes:

1½ cups Cherry Tomatoes
1 teaspoon Extra Virgin Olive Oil

For Topping:

½ teaspoon Lime Zest, grated freshly
½ tablespoon Fresh Lime Juice
1 tablespoon Fresh Parsley, chopped
Sea Salt and Black Pepper, to taste

Directions:

1. For chicken, in a bowl, mix together oil, garlic, lime juice and zest. Add chicken and coat generously. Cover and refrigerate to marinate for about 30 minutes.
2. Preheat the grill to medium heat. Grease the grill grate. Remove chicken from marinade and sprinkle with salt and black pepper. Grill chicken for about 5 minutes per side.
3. Meanwhile preheat the oven to 425 degrees F. Line a roasting pan with foil paper. Place tomatoes in prepared pan in single layer. Drizzle with oil. Roast for about 18 to 20 minutes.
4. On a serving plate place tomatoes and topping ingredients and mix. Top with chicken pieces and serve.

Bell Pepper Fete

The divine combination of bell peppers and red onions goes very well with garlic. This wonderfully simple dish is really delicious. Garnish with lemon zest.

Servings: 2
Preparation Time: 10 minutes
Cooking Time: 10 minutes

---

1 Garlic Clove, minced
2 teaspoons Extra Virgin Olive Oil
1 Small Red Onion, sliced
2 Green Bell Peppers, seeded and cut into thin long strips
1 Red Bell Pepper, seeded and cut into thin long strips
1 Yellow Bell Pepper, seeded and cut into thin long strips
Pinch of Red Pepper Flakes, crushed
Sea Salt and Black Pepper, to taste

Directions:

1. In a skillet, heat oil on medium heat. Add in garlic and allow to sauté for approximately 1 minute.
2. Add onion and bell peppers and season with pinch of red pepper flakes, salt and black pepper according to taste. Cook while stirring occasionally for 8 to 9 minutes.

Spicy Salmon with Broccoli

This is one of the perfect fish dishes which turn simple salmon into a quick and healthy meal. Serve with fresh lime wedges.

Servings: 2
Preparation Time: 20 minutes
Cooking Time: 10 minutes

For Salmon:

1 tablespoon Scallions, chopped finely
2 Garlic Cloves, minced
1 tablespoon Fresh Parsley, chopped
2 tablespoons Fresh Lemon Juice
2 tablespoons Extra Virgin Olive Oil
1 tablespoon Balsamic Vinegar
½ tablespoon Onion Powder
Pinch of Red Pepper Flakes, crushed
Pinch of Cayenne Pepper
Sea Salt and Black Pepper, to taste
2 (4-ounces) Salmon Fillets

For Broccoli:

1 Head Broccoli, cut into florets
1 teaspoon Olive Oil
Pinch of Red Pepper Flakes, crushed
Sea Salt and Black Pepper, to taste

Directions:

1. For fish, in a large bowl, add all ingredients except fish and mix until well combined. Add fish and coat with marinade generously. Cover and refrigerate for about 5 to 6 hours.
2. Preheat the oven to 450 degrees F. Place salmon fillets on broiling sheet. Broil for 5 minutes. Then increase the temperature to 500 degrees F. broil for 5 minutes more.
3. Meanwhile place a steamer basket over a pot of water. Place broccoli in steamer basket. Cover and steam for 4 to 5 minutes on medium-high heat. Drain well. Transfer into a bowl. Drizzle with oil and sprinkle with salt and black pepper.
4. In a serving plate, place salmon with broccoli and serve.

Deluxe Vegetables Stew

This is an absolutely delicious veggies stew. This recipe is a sure fun with seasonal vegetables. Serve with fresh veggie salad.

Servings: 2
Preparation Time: 20 minutes
Cooking Time: 30 minutes

½ tablespoon Coconut Oil
1 Onion, chopped finely
2 Garlic Cloves, minced
1 Medium Stalk Celery, sliced
2 Small Carrots, sliced
1 Small Yellow Bell Pepper, seeded and chopped
1 Small Red Bell Pepper, seeded and chopped
½ tablespoon Dried Oregano
½ teaspoon Ground Cumin
¼ teaspoon Red Pepper Flakes
¼ teaspoon Cayenne Pepper
1 cup Low Sodium Vegetable Broth
1 Zucchini, , sliced
1½ cups Grape Tomatoes, halved
1 sprig Fresh Oregano
2 tablespoons Fresh Lemon Juice
Sea Salt and Black Pepper, to taste

Directions:

1. In a large skillet, heat oil on medium heat. Add onion and sauté for 3 to 4 minutes. Add garlic and sauté for 1 minute more.
2. Add celery, carrot, bell peppers, oregano, cumin and spices and cook while stirring occasionally for about 5 minutes.
3. Add remaining ingredients and bring to a boil. Reduce the heat to medium-low. Simmer for15 to 20 minutes.
4. Remove the oregano sprig and season with salt and black pepper. Serve hot.

– 8 –

DETOX DINNER RECIPES

Beef & Veggie Salad

This is a protein packed salad with healthy nutrient. You may make this filling beef salad for an entrée at dinner or as desired. Top with fresh basil leaves.

Servings: 2
Preparation Time: 20 minutes
Cooking Time: 12 minutes

For Salad:

2 teaspoons Extra Virgin Olive Oil
½ pound Grass Fed Beef Steak
Sea Salt and Black Pepper, to taste
1 cup Bean Sprouts
2 cups Grape Tomatoes, halved
1 English Cucumber, chopped
1 Red Onion, sliced thinly
1 cup Fresh Lettuce Leaves, torn
½ Bunch Coriander Leaves, chopped

½ Bunch Basil Leaves, chopped

For Vinaigrette:

1 Garlic Clove, minced
1 teaspoon Extra Virgin Olive Oil
1 teaspoon Balsamic Vinegar
1 teaspoon Fresh Lime Juice
1 teaspoon Lime Zest, grated freshly
Sea Salt and Black Pepper, to taste

Directions:

1. Preheat the grill to medium. Grease the grill grate.
2. Sprinkle steak with salt and black pepper. Grill for about 6 minutes on each side. Transfer aside to cool slightly. Slice the steak thinly crosswise.
3. Meanwhile in a small bowl, add garlic, oil, vinegar, lime juice, zest, salt and black pepper and beat until well combined.
4. In a large serving bowl, add beef and remaining ingredients. Pour dressing and toss to coat well.

Turkey & Spinach Salad

This is a nice tasting salad with remarkable and simple vinaigrette. Garnish with fresh cilantro leaves.

Servings: 2
Preparation Time: 20 minutes

1/3 cup Low Sodium Vegetable Broth
2 teaspoons Olive Oil
2 teaspoons Dijon Mustard
Sea Salt and Black Pepper, to taste
½ pound Grilled Boneless, Skinless Turkey Breast, cubed
4 cups Baby Spinach Leaves
1 Small Red Bell Pepper, seeded and chopped
1 Scallion, chopped
1 Stalk Celery, chopped

Directions:

1. In a small bowl, add broth, oil, mustard, salt and black pepper and beat until properly combined. Place aside.
2. In a large serving bowl, add all remaining ingredients and mix. Pour vinaigrette and gently, toss to coat well.

Spicy Beef Soup

This hearty soup is great for a cold winter day or any ordinary day. Red pepper adds a spicy kick to it and it is garnish with freshly grated lime zest.

Servings: 4
Preparation Time: 20 minutes
Cooking Time: 1hour 40 minutes

½ tablespoon Olive Oil
1 Medium Onion, chopped
1 Garlic Clove, minced
1 pound Grass Fed Beef Stew Meat, trimmed and cut into bite size pieces
2½ cups Low Sodium Vegetable Broth
1 Celery Stalk, sliced
2 cups Ripe Roma Tomatoes, crushed
1/8 teaspoon Ground Red Pepper
Sea Salt and Black Pepper, to taste
1 Red Bell Pepper, seeded and chopped
1 cup Cabbage, chopped
2 tablespoon Fresh Lime Juice

Directions:

1. In a large soup pan, heat oil on medium heat. Add onion and garlic and sauté for 4 to 5 minutes. Add

beef and cook, stirring for 4 to 5 minutes.

2. Add broth, celery, tomatoes and seasoning and bring to boiling point. Lower the heat to low. Cover and simmer for about 1 hour.
3. Add bell pepper and cabbage and cover and simmer for 25 to 30 minutes.
4. Stir in lime juice and serve.

Tofu & Shrimp Soup

This is a light and flavorful soup. It is uniquely flavored and combines shrimp, tofu and peas very nicely. Drizzle this soup with lime juice.

Servings: 2
Preparation Time: 15 minutes
Cooking Time: 8 minutes

½ tablespoon Olive Oil
½-inch Fresh Ginger Piece, minced
1 Garlic Clove, minced
6-ounces Shrimp, shelled and deveined
1¼ cups Low Sodium Chicken Broth
¼ cup Frozen Peas
½ cup Tofu, drained and chopped
Sea Salt and Black Pepper, to taste

Directions:

1. In a large pan, heat oil on medium heat. Add ginger and garlic and sauté for 1 minute. Add shrimps and sauté for 3 to 4 minutes. Transfer the shrimps in a bowl.
2. Add broth and bring to a boil. Reduce the heat to medium. Add peas, tofu, salt and black pepper and simmer for 2 to 3 minutes. Return the shrimp into

soup and serve.

Medley Cabbage Soup

This is a favorite soup for those want to be slim and trim but it is also a really nourishing and tasty soup. Top with freshly grated lemon zest and enjoy.

Servings: 4
Preparation Time: 15 minutes
Cooking Time: 25 minutes

½ tablespoon Olive Oil
2 Garlic Cloves, minced
1 Medium Onion, chopped
¼ cup Carrot, sliced finely
¼ cup Scallions, chopped
4 cups Low Sodium Vegetable Broth
¼ Head Red Cabbage, chopped coarsely
¼ Head Green Cabbage, chopped coarsely
¼ cup Homemade Tomato Puree
Sea Salt and Black Pepper, to taste

Directions:

1. In a large soup pan, heat oil on medium heat. Add garlic and onion and sauté for 1 to 2 minutes. Add carrot and scallions and sauté for about 3 minutes.
2. Add remaining ingredients and bring to a boil. Reduce the heat to low. Simmer for about 15 to 20

minutes.

Lamb Chops & Herbs

This is a very simple yet impressive recipe for dinner. These well-chosen detox friendly ingredients make this dish impressive and delicious. Serve with steamed baby carrots.

Servings: 2
Preparation Time: 10 minutes
Cooking Time: 8 minutes

1½ tablespoons Olive Oil
3 Garlic Cloves, chopped
½ teaspoons Fresh Thyme, chopped
½ teaspoon Fresh Oregano, chopped
1/8 teaspoon Red Pepper Flakes
Sea Salt and Black Peppers, to taste
½ pound Grass Fed Lamb Chops

Directions:

1. In a food processor, add all ingredients except lamb and pulse until smooth. Transfer the mixture in a bowl. Add lamb chops and coat with the mixture. Cover and refrigerate to marinate for about 8 hours.
2. Preheat the broiler to medium. Place the chops in a baking sheet in a single layer.
3. Broil for about 4 minutes from both sides.

Salmon with Mustard Sauce

The delicacy of herbs with Dijon mustard in this sauce goes very nicely and adds a fantastic taste to the salmon. Serve with fresh lemon wedges.

Servings: 2
Preparation Time: 10 minutes
Cooking Time: 8 minutes

---

2 tablespoons Dijon Mustard
½ tablespoon Olive Oil
1 Garlic Clove, chopped
1/3 teaspoon Fresh Oregano
1/3 teaspoon Fresh Basil
½ tablespoon Fresh Lemon Juice
2 (4-ounces) Salmon Fillets
Sea Salt and Black Pepper, to taste

Directions:

1. In a food processor, add mustard, oil, garlic and fresh herbs and pulse until well combined. Place aside.
2. Preheat the broiler. Line a baking sheet with foil paper and then grease it. Place fish fillets in the prepared baking sheet, then sprinkle with a little sea salt and black pepper according to your taste.
3. Broil for 3 minutes. Flip the side. Place the mustard

sauce over salmon fillets. Broil for 5 minutes more.

Peppery Sautéed Collard Greens

This quick and easy collard greens recipe is also a bit spicy with the red pepper flakes. Top with chopped almonds and enjoy.

Servings: 2
Preparation Time: 10 minutes
Cooking Time: 6 minutes

---

1 tablespoon Olive Oil
4 Garlic Cloves, chopped
1 pound Collard Greens
1 Small Fresh Green Chile, chopped
Sea Salt and Black Pepper, to taste
Pinch of Red Pepper Flakes
½ tablespoon Fresh Lemon Juice

Directions:

1. In a large skillet, heat oil on medium heat. Add in chopped garlic and allow it to sauté for about a minute.
2. Add collard greens and remaining ingredients except lemon juice and sauté for 4 to 5 minutes.
3. Stir in lemon juice and serve hot.

Zesty Haddock with Olives

This recipe is among one of the finest fish recipes with a balanced flavor. Orange adds a refreshing citrus flavor to this baked fish. Serve with chopped scallions.

Servings: 2
Preparation Time: 15 minutes
Cooking Time: 10 minutes

---

2 (4-ounces) Haddock Fillets
1 tablespoon Olive Oil, divided
2 tablespoons Fresh Lime Juice
1 teaspoon Orange Zest, grated freshly
Sea Salt and Black Pepper, to taste
1 Small Shallot, chopped
1 Large Orange, peeled, seeded and cut into segments
2 tablespoons Black Olives, pitted and halved
2 tablespoons Fresh Rosemary, chopped

Directions:

1. In a bowl, add fish, 1 teaspoon of oil, orange juice and zest and mix well. Keep aside for 15 minutes. Preheat the oven to 400 degrees F.
2. In an oven proof skillet, heat remaining oil on medium heat. Remove fish from marinade and reserve the marinade. Add fish in skillet and sprinkle

with salt and black pepper. Cook for about 3 minutes. Flip the side and add shallots. Cook for 1 minute more.

3. Add reserved marinade, half of orange segments and olives in skillet. Top with rosemary. Transfer the skillet in oven. Bake for about 6 minutes.

4. In a serving plate, place fish fillets with sauce mixture from skillet. Top with remaining orange segments and serve.

Turkey with Mushrooms

This is a delicious and healthy recipe for the whole family. The flavor of this dish is hearty and earthy. Garnish with chopped scallions.

Servings: 2
Preparation Time: 15 minutes
Cooking Time: 35 minutes

½ pound Boneless Turkey Breast Tenderloins
½ tablespoon Olive Oil
¼ teaspoon Dried Rosemary, crushed
3 tablespoons Low Sodium Vegetable Broth
Smoked Paprika, to taste
Sea Salt and Black Pepper, to taste
½ cup Button Mushrooms, sliced

Directions:

1. Preheat the oven to 375 degrees F. Grease a baking dish.
2. Place turkey tenderloins in prepared baking dish. Drizzle with oil. In a bowl, mix together remaining ingredients except mushrooms. Pour mixture over tenderloins evenly. Place mushrooms around tenderloins evenly.
3. Bake for 30 to 35 minutes.

Spicy Beef with Spinach

This is a fantastic for a delicious family dinner. This healthy dish is topped with chopped almonds.

Servings: 2
Preparation Time: 15 minutes
Cooking Time: 30 minutes

---

1 tablespoon Olive Oil
1 Medium Onion, sliced finely
1 Garlic Clove, chopped
1 Green Chile Pepper, sliced thinly
½ teaspoon Ground Cumin
½ teaspoon Ground Coriander
1/8 teaspoon Chili Powder
¼ teaspoon Ground Turmeric
½ pound Grass Fed Beef Tenderloin, cubed
Sea Salt, to taste
½ cup Unsweetened Coconut Milk
½ cup Roma Tomatoes, chopped
½ pound Fresh Spinach, torn
1 teaspoon Fresh Lemon Juice

Directions:

1. In a large skillet, heat oil on medium heat. Next, add in onion and garlic and sauté for 5 minutes. Add Chile

pepper and sauté for 2 to 3 minutes. Add spices and sauté for about 2 minutes.

2. Add beef and season with salt and cook for about 3 minutes. Add coconut milk and tomatoes and bring to a boil. Reduce the heat to low. Cover and simmer for about 15 to 20 minutes while stirring often.

3. Add spinach and cook uncovered for 5 minutes more or until thickens. Stir in lemon juice and serve hot.

Baked Chicken with Brussels Sprouts

This is a yummy dinner recipe and may be great for the weekend. Your whole family may enjoy this meal. Top with crushed rosemary.

Servings: 2
Preparation Time: 15 minutes
Cooking Time: 1 hour 5 minutes

½ tablespoon Olive Oil
2 (4-ounces) Boneless, Skinless Chicken Breasts
½ pound Brussels sprouts
1½ tablespoons Fresh Thyme Leaves
¾ cup White Onion, chopped
1 cup Low Sodium Vegetable Broth
Sea Salt and Black Pepper, to taste
1/8 teaspoon Red Chili Powder

Directions:

1. Preheat the oven to 375 degrees Fahrenheit then lightly grease a baking dish.
2. In a skillet, heat oil on medium heat. Add chicken and cook for 4 to 5 minutes or until browned evenly.
3. Place chicken in prepared baking dish. Arrange Brussels sprouts around chicken breasts. Top with thyme and onion. Pour broth and add in salt, pepper

and red pepper flakes. Cover and bake for 20 minutes.

4. Increase the temperature to 400 degrees F. Uncover and bake for 30 to 40 minutes more.

Sautéed Snow Peas Summer

This is one of the super quick and easy recipes for a light dinner. This is a colorful dish which has a beautiful presentation. Garnish with freshly grated lemon zest.

Servings: 2
Preparation Time: 15 minutes
Cooking Time: 5 minutes

---

2 teaspoons Olive Oil
1 Garlic Clove, minced
2 cups Snow Peas, trimmed
3 tablespoons Water
12 to 14 Grape Tomatoes, halved
Sea Salt and Black Pepper, to taste
Pinch of Cayenne Pepper

Directions:

1. In a skillet, heat oil on medium heat. Next, add in garlic and sauté for approximately 1 minute.
2. Add snow peas and water and cook for about 2 minutes or until all liquid is absorbed. Add tomatoes and cook for about 2 minutes more.
3. Stir in salt, black pepper and cayenne pepper and remove from heat. Serve hot.

Beef with Bok Choy

This is a wonderful dish with the combo of beef and bok choy. It is really flavorful in taste. Serve with a topping of freshly chopped basil.

Servings: 2
Preparation Time: 10 minutes
Cooking Time: 15 minutes

½ pound Grass Fed Steak, trimmed and cubed
Sea Salt to taste
1 teaspoon Ground Cumin
2 teaspoons Olive Oil
1 tablespoon Garlic, minced
2 cups Bok Choy, sliced thinly
½ cup Low Sodium Vegetable Broth
Black Pepper, to taste
Pinch of Cayenne Pepper

Directions:

1. Coat beef steak with salt and cumin evenly. In a skillet, heat oil on medium-high heat. Add beef and cook for 3 to 4 minutes. Transfer into a plate and cover with a foil paper.
2. In the same skillet, add garlic and sauté for about 1 minute. Add bok choy and seasoning and stir fry for 1

to 2 minutes. Add broth and bring to boiling point. Lower the heat to medium and continue to cook for about 3 to 4 minutes.

3. Add beef and increase the heat to medium. Cook while stirring occasionally for about 3 to 4 minutes.

Chicken with Steamed Veggies

This chicken recipe is delicious, healthy, and quite easy to prepare. It is a good way to have your kids to their veggies. Serve with fresh lime wedges.

Servings: 2
Preparation Time: 10 minutes
Cooking Time: 16 minutes

½ pound Asparagus, julienned
½ pound Snap Beans, trimmed
3 teaspoons Olive Oil, divided
2 (4-ounces) Boneless, Skinless Chicken Breasts, pounded to ¼-inch thickness
Sea Salt and Black Pepper, to taste
1 cup Low Sodium Vegetable Broth
2 teaspoons Olive Oil
1 tablespoon Fresh Lemon Juice
½ teaspoon Fresh Lemon Zest, grated freshly
1 tablespoon Fresh Parsley, chopped

Directions:

1. Place a steamer basket over a pot of water. Place asparagus and beans in steamer basket. Cover and steam for 4 to 5 minutes on medium-high heat. Drain well. Transfer into a bowl.

2. In a large skillet, heat 1½ teaspoons oil on medium heat. Add chicken and cook for 2 to 3 minutes per side. Transfer the chicken in a plate and cover with foil paper.
3. Add broth and cook for about 5 to 6 minutes. Add remaining oil and remaining ingredients and cook, stirring continuously for about 2 minutes. Remove from heat.
4. In a serving plate, place chicken and steamed veggies. Top with sauce and serve.

Sautéed Beef with Bell Peppers

This sautéed beef is easy to make and really tasty and full of nutrients. Serve with a garnish of chopped scallions.

Servings: 2
Preparation Time: 10 minutes
Cooking Time: 10 minutes

---

1 tablespoon Olive Oil
1 Garlic Clove, minced
½ pound Grass Fed Lean Ground Beef
¼ cup Red Onion, chopped
¼ cup Red Bell Pepper, seeded and chopped
¼ cup Green Bell Pepper, seeded and chopped
Sea Salt and Black Pepper, to taste

Directions:

1. In a large skillet, heat oil on medium-high heat. Next, add in garlic and sauté for 1 minute.
2. Add beef and sauté for 3 to 4 minutes. Add onion and bell peppers and sauté for 4 to 5 minutes.
3. Season with salt and black pepper and serve hot.

Shrimp Veggie Medley

This recipe features a healthy and tasty twist to simple shrimp dishes. Serve with fresh lemon slices.

Servings: 2
Preparation Time: 20 minutes
Cooking Time: 18 minutes

½ pound Shrimp, shelled and deveined
1 tablespoon Balsamic Vinegar
1 tablespoon Fresh Lime Juice
1½ tablespoons Olive Oil, divided
1 Small White Onion, cut into wedges
½ cup Crimini Mushrooms, sliced
¾ cup Cabbage, chopped
1 Small Red Bell Pepper, seeded and cubed
1-inch Fresh Ginger Piece, grated finely
¼ pound Snow Peas, trimmed

Directions:

1. In a bowl, add shrimp, vinegar, lime juice and ½ tablespoon of oil and mix well. Place aside for about 10 minutes. Remove shrimp from marinade and reserve the marinade.
2. In a large skillet, heat remaining oil on medium-high heat. Next, add in shrimp and allow to cook for

approximately 2 minutes on both sides. Transfer shrimp into a bowl.

3. Add onion and sauté for about 5 minutes. Add mushrooms and sauté for 2 minutes. Add cabbage and bell peppers and sauté for about 3 to 4 minutes. Add ginger and snow peas and sauté for about 1 minute.

4. Add shrimp and reserved marinade and cook for about 3 to 4 minutes or until sauce is thickened to your preference.

Stir Fried Tofu Broccoli Bowl

This recipe gives tofu a nice and delish texture. Tofu and broccoli stir fry is a tasty dish that you can easily prepare for dinner.

Servings: 2
Preparation Time: 15 minutes
Cooking Time: 20 minutes

¾ pound Broccoli, cut into bite sized pieces
1 tablespoon Olive Oil
8-ounces firm Tofu, drained and cubed
¼ cup Low Sodium Vegetable Broth
1 tablespoon Balsamic Vinegar
2 Garlic Cloves, minced
1/8 teaspoon Red Pepper Flakes
¼ cup Walnuts, toasted and chopped

Directions:

1. In a pan of boiling salted water, add broccoli and cook for approximately 2-3 minutes. Drain the broccoli and place aside.
2. In a large skillet, heat oil on medium heat. Add tofu and cook for 10 to 15 minutes, turning once. Transfer the tofu into a bowl, lined with paper towel.
3. Meanwhile in a bowl, mix together remaining ingredients except walnuts. In the same skillet, add

broccoli and increase the temperature to high heat. Cook, stirring occasionally for about 2 to 3 minute. Add sauce in skillet and cook for 2 to 3 minutes or until just start to thicken.

4. Stir in tofu and cook for about 1 to 2 minutes.

Chicken with Tomatoes & Asparagus

This is an amazingly delicious recipe. Surely you may want to make this dish again and again. Serve with a little drizzle of lime juice or as desired.

Servings: 2
Preparation Time: 15 minutes
Cooking Time: 35 minutes

---

1 tablespoon Olive Oil
2 (4-ounces) Skinless Chicken Thighs
½ teaspoon Dried Thyme crushed
Sea Salt and Black Pepper, to taste
Pinch of Red Pepper Flakes, crushed
Garlic Powder, to taste
Onion Powder, to taste
1 cup Cherry Tomatoes
½ Bunch Asparagus, trimmed
1 tablespoon Fresh Oregano, chopped

Directions:

1. Preheat the oven to 400 degrees F.
2. In an oven proof skillet, heat oil on medium-high heat. Add chicken thighs and sprinkle with dried thyme and seasonings. Cook for 5 minutes per side. Transfer chicken into a plate.

3. Place tomatoes, asparagus and oregano in the same skillet. Sprinkle with salt and black pepper. Place chicken thighs on top.
4. Roast for about 20 to 25 minutes.

Vegan Lamb Chops

These tasty and succulent lamb chops are perfect for making a midweek dinner with the addition delicious veggies. Enjoy.

Servings: 2
Preparation Time: 15 minutes
Cooking Time: 25 minutes

2 tablespoons Olive Oil, divided
½ pound Grass Fed Lamb Chops
Sea Salt and Black Pepper, to taste
3 Artichoke Hearts, cut into wedges
1 Medium White Onion, sliced thinly
½ cup Grape Tomatoes, halved
1¼ cups Low Sodium Vegetable Broth
¼ cup Black Olives, pitted and halved
½ tablespoon Lemon Zest, freshly grated

Directions:

1. In a large skillet, heat oil on medium heat. Add chops and sprinkle with salt and black pepper, to taste. Cook for 4 to 5 minutes from both sides. Transfer into a bowl and cover with a foil paper to keep it warm.
2. In the same skillet, heat remaining oil on medium heat. Add artichokes and onion and cook for 4 to 5

minutes. Add tomatoes and broth. Cover and cook for 4 to 5 minutes. Uncover and cook for 4 to 5 minutes more.

3. Stir in olives and lemon zest. Season with salt and black pepper and remove from heat.

4. In a serving plate, place veggie mixture. Top with chops and serve.

Cauliflower Salmon Surprise

This salmon and cauliflower recipe may surprise you. With a simple sprinkling of sea salt and pepper it really tastes delicious. Serve with fresh slices of lemon or as desired.

Servings: 2
Preparation Time: 15 minutes
Cooking Time: 25 minutes

---

1 pound Cauliflower Florets, cut into ½-inch slices
2 tablespoons Olive Oil, divided
Sea Salt and Black Pepper, to taste
2 (4-ounces) Salmon Fillets
½ tablespoon Balsamic Vinegar
½ tablespoon Fresh Thyme, minced
½ tablespoon Fresh Rosemary, minced

Directions:

1. Preheat the broiler and place rack 6-inches away from heating element. Next, line a baking sheet with foil paper. Place cauliflower on prepared baking sheet in single layer. Drizzle with 1 tablespoon oil and sprinkle with salt and black pepper. Broil for about 10 minutes.
2. In a bowl, add fish. Drizzle with remaining oil and sprinkle with salt and black pepper. Remove baking

sheet from oven. Place fish fillets over cauliflower, skin side up. Broil for about 6 to 7 minutes.

3. Remove from oven and place fish and cauliflower in a serving plate. Drizzle with vinegar. Top with fresh herbs and serve.

– 9 –

ESSENTIAL DETOX FOODS SHOPPING LIST

Here is a helpful guide of typically healthy detox foods for your shopping list.

1. **Healthy Proteins** such as: sardines, shrimp, wild salmon and canned salmon, tofu, herring, chicken, grass-fed meat, canned salmon, sardines or herring, tempeh, hard boiled eggs
2. **Non-starchy Vegetables** such as: cabbage, turnip, bok choy, broccoli, lettuce, mushroom, squash, cauliflower, cucumber, tomatoes, bell peppers, celery, onions, asparagus, dandelion greens, zucchini, kale, spinach, snow peas, green beans, jalapeno peppers, shallots, mixed greens, arugula, artichoke, Swiss chard, mustard greens, radicchio, chives tomatoes, bean sprouts, eggplant, onions, turnip greens, beet greens, endive, parsley, watercress, fennel, radishes, garlic, Brussels sprouts, ginger root, snap beans, collard greens and hearts of palm.
3. **Healthy Nuts** such as: walnuts, almonds, pecans
4. **Healthy Seeds** such as: chia seeds, flaxseeds, pumpkin seeds, sunflower seeds and sesame seeds
5. **Healthy Fats** such as: extra-virgin olive oil and coconut oil and avocado

6. **Healthy Sugars** such as: low sugar fruits including limes, pumpkin, lemons and berries
7. **Healthy Vinegars**: apple cider vinegar, balsamic vinegar
8. **Natural Detox and Organic Herbs, Seasonings and Spices**: stick to homemade, gluten-free and low-sugar items such as: low-sodium vegetable broth, thyme, rosemary, Dijon mustard, black pepper, chili powder, cumin, sage, cinnamon, coriander, oregano, onion powder, turmeric, cayenne, cilantro, paprika and parsley
9. **Healthy Beverages** such as: filtered water, organic unsweetened coconut milk and organic unsweetened almond milk.
10. **Salt**: regular sea salt

— 10 —

IT'S ALL GOOD!

All in all, detox is a wonderful thing and we should all be doing it from time to time. No longer should you see detoxing as a scheduled event for springtime or the New Year, but you should see it as a way of helping your body to naturally detoxify on a daily basis.

With this cookbook's simple principles and procedures, you will be able to successfully create healthy and flavorful detox meals that will contribute to your healthy lifestyle goals. Many people have experienced significant weight loss and health improvements while eating these recipes during and after a properly structured detox program. Ideally, I strongly believe that we need to rest and cleanse our guts from time to time. From my experience with these recipes, I can confidently say that the health results are simply invaluable.

Thank you for choosing my book. If you find this book to be helpful, I would appreciate if you would let other readers know about it by leaving a book review. I hereby wish you all the best in your quest to detoxify your body, lose weight and experience restored health.

Yours in health,
Sara

Made in the USA
San Bernardino, CA
07 August 2014